Low Thyroid Diet

How to Naturally Treat your Hypothyroidism
by Eating Good and Avoiding Bad Foods

By

Anna Keating

Low Thyroid Diet: How to Naturally Treat your Hypothyroidism by Eating Good and Avoiding Bad Foods

ISBN-10: 1549989995

ISBN-13: 978-1549989995

Warning and Disclaimer

Publisher contact

Skinny Bottle Publishing

books@skinnybottle.com

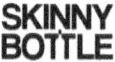

About the author

After having a near-death experience due to an organ failure, Anna Keating promised that she would take a better care of herself. 20 years later, she is a mother of three healthy children and a health advocate who helps others avoid the complications she went through.

Sharing her knowledge and experience with the rest of the world, Anna has a lot to say about our overall health. If you want to avoid health complications due to unhealthy lifestyle and imbalanced diet, then you have come to the right place.

Now What?

Leaving your doctor's office knowing that you are hypothyroid may not be something to be happy about, however, hypothyroidism is not exactly a death sentence. Whether it was you who has been diagnosed or you know someone that struggles with an underactive thyroid, one thing is certain, buying this book was definitely a choice that you will benefit from.

The educational journey that you are about to take through this book will not only give you answers to your questions about why and how does the thyroid stop functioning properly, how to diagnose and treat it, but it will also make you adopt a new lifestyle and diet that will be super friendly to your thyroid hormones and will boost their production.

Providing you with a full and carefully created 21-day hypothyroid meal plan, it is safe to say that this book is the most comprehensive hypothyroidism book you will ever read.

Want to clarify the confusions that were stirred by the conflicting theories online? Join me on this educational ride and permanently treat your hypothyroidism the most natural way.

The Thyroid's Function

Most of us are well aware that there is something called a *thyroid* in our bodies, but also equally unaware of why exactly we have one. If you have bought this book for educational purposes only, you should pay a good attention to this chapter. People usually start appreciating this gland when something goes wrong, so in order to prevent that from happening you will need a good understanding of what the thyroid does for your body.

If you actually struggle with thyroid problems, please do not skip this chapter. It is of great importance that you know the exact thyroid's function if you want to boost and rebalance it.

Before I jump to the medical side of this chapter, I want you to imagine something. Imagine your body as a complex factory. A factory with many machines, moving parts, and workers who operate them. In this complex factory, you can find your thyroid operating as a manager. Without this gland assigning work to workers and telling them what they should do, the work wouldn't get done, or at least not in the proper way.

And while the thyroid isn't exactly the big cheese in this factory – it's 'boss' is the pituitary gland who answers to the hypothalamus (a part of the brain) – we cannot deny the fact that it plays a major part in keeping the balance in the factory. In order for your body to function properly, the thyroid has to be able to 'boss around' other bodily parts.

But, where is the thyroid's office? The thyroid is located at the base of your neck (in the throat), just below the larynx, or otherwise known as the 'voicebox', and in front of the trachea, or also known as the 'windpipe'. It is about 2-inches long and it has a butterfly-like shape. Its two 'wings' are curled around your windpipe, connected by a strip of isthmus (a thyroid tissue). Some people, however, do not have isthmus and their thyroid has two separate lobes.

The thyroid may weigh less than an ounce, but when it comes to your health, it can really pack a wallop. It is a part of the endocrine system, the place where glands produce, store, and release all sorts of hormones into the bloodstream. Think of the endocrine system like the orchestra. In order to play a beautiful symphony, everyone that plays in the orchestra has to do its job efficiently. The thyroid job in the endocrine 'orchestra' is to use the iodine that you consume with food to produce two different hormones:

1.   Triiodothyronine or T3

2.   Thyroxine or T4

The thyroid's hormones are of great importance for our overall health because they keep the metabolism balanced, meaning that they control the way in which our body uses energy. The thyroid's hormones do this by increasing the metabolism of carbs, protein, and fats, which is done by increasing mitochondria, along with many different processes, which are in charge of utilizing these energy products. When the body's usage of carbs, fats, and protein is enhanced, the body temperature and its basal metabolic rate are also increased.

Once the thyroid releases its hormones T3 and T4 in the bloodstream, they start their journey to the body cells. They stop at each and every cell to check if they need some more nutrients or oxygen. If they do then the hormones will step up the metabolism rate, if not, they can also slow it down.

The thyroid hormones are in charge of controlling some vital functions such as:

-      Heart rate

- Breathing

- Muscle strength

- Central and peripheral nervous systems

- Cholesterol levels

- Body temperature

- Body weight

- Menstrual cycles

They also take part in the proper usage of vitamins, affect the adrenaline, as well as help with many different processes. Not to make this list super lengthy, I believe you get the meaning that the thyroid is pretty important gland in the body.

But that is not all. The thyroid is not only made of follicular cells but also has *parafollicular cells* that are in charge of producing the hormone calcitonin. It also has 4 tiny glands called parathyroid glands that are embedded in the thyroid back, and produce the parathyroid hormone. The parathyroid hormone and the calcitonin are also very important for our health because when they work in tandem, they actually keep the calcium levels in check.

What is Hypothyroidism?

It is of great importance that there is a balance between the hormones and the glands in the brain, meaning that the T3 and T4 hormones shouldn't be too low or too high. It is up to the pituitary gland and the hypothalamus to make everything run as clockwork. They are in constant communication and maintain the balance between these two hormones.

The hypothalamus is in charge of producing TRS (THS Releasing Hormones), which signals the pituitary gland to nudge the thyroid to produce either less or more of the hormone, which is done by either decreasing or increasing the thyroid stimulating hormone (THS).

It is simple actually. If there are low T3 and T4 hormones in the bloodstream, the pituitary gland will produce more of the TSH, to tell the thyroid that it should produce more hormones. If the hormones are high, the TSH is decreased so that the thyroid gland can know it should decrease the production of T3 and T4.

Bu in some cases, these glands and hormones cannot exactly work as smooth as a clockwork. In some cases, the thyroid gland just won't do what is it told and continues producing more or fewer hormones than necessary. When that happens, our health is compromised.

If the thyroid works harder than necessary, more T3 and T4 hormones are produced. This condition, when the thyroid produces hormones too enthusiastically is called *hyperthyroidism*. This can happen for a number of reasons, but the most common one that makes the thyroid work overtime is Grave's disease.

There are a number of symptoms that can indicate that there are excessive thyroid hormones in the bloodstream. Hyperthyroidism can cause an increased appetite, but at the same time a sudden weight loss as well. It can lead to rapid and irregular heartbeat or even a pounding heart. When the thyroid is wacky you can become very sensitive to heat, have an itchy and flushed skin, and start sweating excessively. You may experience tremor in your hands which can lead to anxiety, difficulty sleeping, be irritable and nervous, etc. You will also notice hair loss or thinning, muscle weakness, and the list just goes on.

Some of these symptoms may be more dangerous than others, but nevertheless, if a person experiences a few of these symptoms, it is of utmost importance that the thyroid gland gets checked for hyperthyroidism. If left untreated, hyperthyroidism can take a toll on people's health, making them lose bone density and seriously increasing the risk of stroke.

If hyperthyroidism is on one side of the coin, the hypothyroidism is on the other. Hypothyroidism – the condition that we will focus on in this book – happens when the thyroid is underactive and produces fewer hormones than the body needs in order to have a balanced metabolism.

Think of the thyroid hormones like the heat and the thyroid gland as the heater. If it is cold in the room, you would expect your heater to do its job and warm you up. If it doesn't work properly you will be cold. When there are an insufficient amount of thyroid hormones in the body, the thyroid gland is supposed to produce more. If it is unable to do so, the lack of hormones can disrupt the balance within the body and negatively affect our health.

The fact that you do not hear about hypothyroidism enough does not mean that there are not that many hypothyroid people, but that most of the people that are, have no clue about it. The estimates obviously vary and we cannot possibly know the exact number, however, there are approximately 10 million people in the US only, that are affected by this condition. According to the American Thyroid Association, 12 percent of the overall American population will develop a serious thyroid condition at some point, while up to 40 percent will suffer from some level of underactive thyroid. The most susceptible group of people for developing this condition are women, especially those that are older. Those who have autoimmune diseases such as celiac disease, type 1 diabetes, or rheumatoid arthritis are also at high risk for developing hypothyroidism.

What Causes It?

If you have been diagnosed with hypothyroidism or fear that you have an underactive thyroid, it is important to know the common causes of this condition so that you can pinpoint exactly what was the reason for your thyroid to produce (or may produce) fewer thyroid hormones that your body needs for normal functioning.

Remember, these are only the most common causes. There are high chances that the reason why your thyroid is not working properly can be found on this list, but that doesn't necessarily have to be the case. Your hypothyroidism may be caused by something else entirely. It is best to consult it with your doctor who knows your unique medical history and can give a more accurate response to what causes your hypothyroidism.

Hashimoto's Thyroiditis

In developed countries, the most common cause of hypothyroidism is the autoimmune condition called Hashimoto's thyroiditis. Hashimoto's thyroiditis is an autoimmune endocrine disorder that happens when the thyroid gland gets inflamed.

There are nearly 10 million people affected by this disorder in the US alone. 10 percent of the women who are over 30 have Hashimoto's thyroiditis, and it is important to mention that this disease affects women more than it affects men.

So how and why exactly does Hashimoto's thyroiditis occur? Hashimoto's thyroiditis, like I said, is characterized by the present thyroid inflammation. When a person has this disorder, his body begins to produce antibodies that it will attack itself with, in order to destroy the thyroid gland. I know how you may think that this doesn't make any sense at all, but the truth is, all of this happens because the immune system is mistaken. Thinking mistakenly that the cells of the thyroid gland are not actually a part of the body, the body does its best to destroy them before they can harm it by causing serious damage or illness. Of course, this isn't true, but since the immune system thinks it is, the only thing it can do is play for defense.

That defense causes the thyroid's tissue to decay gradually and eventually results in victory for the immune system, meaning that the thyroid gland will no longer be able to produce needed hormones. That condition is hypothyroidism.

Medical experts believe that nearly 90 percent of people with hypothyroidism also suffer from Hashimoto's thyroiditis, however, this is surely not the only thing that can cause this condition.

Poor Diet

Just like with almost any other condition, poor diet that lacks in nutrient-rich foods can also be blamed for the occurrence of hypothyroidism. If your diet is not rich in the trace minerals iodine and selenium – which are essential for the normal thyroid function – you are at high risk of developing thyroid disorders. Your thyroid needs these nutrients in order to produce the necessary amount of hormones. But that is not the only reason why iodine and selenium are super important for your thyroid. The thing is, they also play a major protective role. For instance, a selenium deficiency can stop the activity of glutathione, a very powerful antioxidant that fights oxidative stress and is in charge of controlling inflammation. The disrupted glutathione function can also lead to thyroiditis.

Hormone Imbalance

Although not that common, the thyroidal problems don't have to occur in the thyroid itself. In some rare cases, the hypothyroidism has actually more to do not with the thyroid, but the gland that controls it – which is the pituitary gland. Some problems that happen in the pituitary may disrupt its production of the simulating hormones THS. That negative impact on the pituitary will give the thyroid inaccurate signals, meaning that the thyroid will not get the proper simulations needed for the adequate production of the T3 and T4 hormones, which will obviously lead to thyroid disorders.

Medications

There are some medications that can cause a change in the thyroid function and contribute to the development of hypothyroidism:

Amiodarone – This medication is used to treat heart rhythm disorders, but thanks to its high iodine content, amiodarone can cause hypothyroidism in about 5-20 percent of the patients that take this medication regularly. The high iodine levels in this medication can result in hypothyroidism by inhibiting the release of the thyroid hormones, as well as the conversion of the T3 and T4 hormones. If you are confused by how iodine can harm the thyroid since we said that it is super helpful, let me put it simply; only the proper amount of iodine can be beneficial for your metabolism. Too much or too little iodine can actually cause the thyroid to stop working correctly.

Lithium – Treating depression and bipolar disorders, this medication can actually slow the production, as well as the release of the thyroid hormones. This is not at all insignificant since nearly 20-30 percent of the patients that have been prescribed regular lithium dosage are known to develop hypothyroidism.

Anti-Thyroid Medications – If you have an overactive thyroid gland which produces more hormones than necessary (known as hyperthyroidism), your doctor may prescribe you some anti-thyroid medications to slow down the production and release of T3 and T4 hormones. However, you need to be very careful and follow the exact dosage, since high doses of these medications will not treat your hyperthyroidism, but help you develop its opponent – hypothyroidism.

Interleukin-2 (IL-2) – Patients suffering from leukemia and metastatic cancers may be prescribed with Interleukin-2. They may be helpful with their conditions, however, it has been proven that approximately 2 percent of them end up with hypothyroidism.

Interferon-Alpha – Although this is not that significant, it is not right to left it unmentioned. Patients suffering from malignant tumors, as well as those who have been diagnosed with hepatitis B and C are usually prescribed with this medications. As a result, a small percentage of them end up with thyroid dysfunctions such as hypothyroidism.

Gut Inflammation

Although an unhealthy gut may not seem that dangerous to you, it can, in fact, leave you nutrient deficient and support the body's autoimmune activity. Gut inflammation (leaky gut syndrome) can be caused by allergies, food sensitivities, elevated stress levels, bacterial imbalances, etc. When leaky gut invades your body, tiny particles from your gut leak out into the bloodstream through cracks and small openings in the gut lining, which created the autoimmune flow followed by other negative symptoms and conditions (such as hypothyroidism).

Problems with the Thyroid

Other problems with the thyroid can lead to its insufficient production of hormones. For instance, if your thyroid has been removed surgically, it is obvious that you are about to develop hypothyroidism. In that case, the doctors will prescribe medications that will replace the T3 and T4 hormones immediately after the surgery to prevent you from experiencing the negative symptoms.

Also, this condition can be developed in rare cases when people are born without a thyroid (thyroid agenesis), as well as in cases of radioactive iodine destruction of the thyroid – a common therapy for treating hyperthyroidism and thyroid cancer.

Sarcoidosis

It is also common for abnormal growths to invade the thyroid and take the place of this gland's healthy tissues. Sarcoidosis is an autoimmune disorder where inflamed tissues form throughout the body. When sarcoidosis is present it can easily replace the healthy thyroid tissues with inflamed tissues, inhibiting the production of the thyroid hormones, which will, in turn, result in hypothyroidism.

Genetics

Although this condition is not very common, there are some cases where infants are born with a dysfunctional thyroid gland, which is a genetic condition that is called congenital hypothyroidism. And while there is evidence that shows that people have more chances of developing hypothyroidism if they have a close family member who has struggled with autoimmune diseases, the NIH (National Institute of Health) says that the chances for a newborn to be born with congenital hypothyroidism are pretty low, or 1 in 4000 to be exact.

Emotional Stress

Stress can pretty much take a toll on every single aspect of our health, and the thyroid function is not an exception. It has a strong negative impact on our hormones and it is known to have the power to worsen inflammation. By raising the levels of cortisol and adrenaline, stress can disrupt the neurotransmitter function and negatively affect the thyroid function.

Inactivity

You know how exercise and regular activity are important for our health? Well, the same way being sedentary can do just the opposite. Since physical activity plays a major part in controlling stress and managing the hormonal function in the brain, you can only imagine what happens to out hormones when we lack exercise. Many studies have confirmed that regular activity manages stress, supports better sleep, and help you maintain a healthy weight, all of which reduce the risk of hypothyroidism. If you lack it, however, the risk of this condition is increased.

Pregnancy

Although there is no actual answer as to why this happens, some women tend to produce a high thyroid hormone content that is followed by a rapid decline, during or right after pregnancy. This hormonal condition is called postpartum thyroiditis. Although in most cases these symptoms disappear after 12-18 months after giving birth, for some women they result in permanent hypothyroidism.

Detecting Hypothyroidism

Did you know that the thyroid is actually known as the 'master gland'? The thyroid has not only earned this title because of its super important role of producing essential hormones, but also because of its ability to help convert nutrients from food into usable energy. Also, the hormones produced by the thyroid can assist the liver in breaking down cholesterol, as well as simulate those enzymes that are required for controlling the triglyceride levels.

Since the thyroid gland plays such an important part in our metabolism, and a balanced metabolism is crucial for our health, you can only imagine how noticeable and widespread the problems caused by the lack of thyroid hormones can really be. That is why it is of utmost importance to detect hypothyroidism in time, so you can take the next steps towards the right treatment.

Symptoms

If you have an underactive thyroid, your metabolism will show it. It will soon become sluggish and slow. This will not only slow you down by constantly making you feel tired or push you to a never-ending struggle to lose weight, but it will also result in moodiness. Since your mood is definitely the first thing that gets attacked when there is a change in your hormone levels, you can only imagine the mental symptoms that are associated with hypothyroidism. The thyroid plays an important role in regulating the neurotransmitters that control your emotions and the signaling of nerves, so drastic emotional changes when you have unbalanced thyroid hormones, are only expected.

Not to exhaust you with the lengthy list of all of the possible symptoms that one can experience as a result of hypothyroidism, these are the most common symptoms reported by the majority of hypothyroid patients:

-       Fatigue

-       Goiter (nodules found at the back of the neck that are sometimes accompanied by coughing, tightness or swelling of the throat)

-       Hair loss

-       Constipation

-       Weight gain

-       Anxiety

-       Depression

-       Rough and cracked skin

-       Tenderness and aches in the muscles

-       Trouble breathing

-       Menstrual cycle changes

-       Frequent flu and cold

-       Swelling and stiffness in the joints

-       Feeling cold

-       Decreased libido

-       Memory loss

- Jaundice (present in severe cases)

- Tongue size increase (present in severe cases)

- Slowed speech (present in severe cases)

Know that you don't have to experience every single one of those symptoms to have hypothyroidism. Just like everyone is different and reacts differently to different disorders, the same way there are different versions of hypothyroidism. For instance, you may be more affected with memory loss, fatigue, and depression, while other patients may have hair loss, cracked skin, and constipation.

It is actually the thyroid stimulating hormone (THS) that has an effect on the severity of this disorder. For instance, if you have a mild form of hypothyroidism and a low level of TSH, the chances of you not noticing – or even not having any – symptoms, are pretty high. That is mainly because the hormone levels still haven't dropped to an alarming level that can have a significant negative impact on your metabolism. The more this condition progresses, the more symptoms you will notice.

Mild hypothyroidism is considered to be the early stage of this disorder. It can progress to full-blown hypothyroidism if lifestyle changes and hypothyroidism diet are not adopted from the beginning. This can, of course, worsen the problems and lead to numerous complications.

In some cases where the hypothyroidism is extremely severe, the patients can fall into a myxedema coma, which is a condition in which the person can have a declines mental status, experience hypothermia, and even the slowing of the internal organs. If you or the person you know that has hypothermia begins showing stupor or lethargy, an emergency medical help must be sought.

Although the myxedema coma is generally rare, it can happen to those patients who had a severe hypothyroidism and were not aware of it, or intentionally left it untreated. It is mostly elderly women that fall into myxedema coma, and usually during the winter months.

Another symptom that you should know about is the thyroid nodules, which are basically a cell buildup inside the thyroid that can create an abnormal lump or growth. And while most of these nodules are not that dangerous, some of them have the tendency to become cancerous over a certain period of time.

Diagnosing Hypothyroidism

It is important to know that there are also other conditions that may share a few symptoms with the hypothyroidism, so do not think that you have successfully diagnosed yourself after checking a few symptoms from the list found in this book. You are not a doctor. In order for you to be or not be diagnosed with hypothyroidism, you need to pay your doctor a visit.

Hypothyroidism can only be diagnosed by a physician. This is usually done by an endocrinologist, but in some obvious cases, the prime doctor can also evaluate and diagnose this condition.

The diagnose can only be reached after a thorough review of physical examination, symptoms, medical history, risk factors, and most importantly, a blood test.

Symptoms

Like I said, the symptoms should be merely a sign that you need to consult with your physician. No condition can be accurately diagnosed by symptoms alone, and neither can hypothyroidism. Many of the symptoms of hypothyroidism are also common complaints by many people. For instance, just because you have been experiencing anxiety, memory loss, hair loss, and weight gain, doesn't mean that you have an underactive thyroid. You may be dealing with a difficult time that makes you eat more hence gain weight, be anxious, lose concentration hence memory loss, and the hair loss can also be a result of excessive stress. Your doctor will go through the symptoms you have been experiencing with you and ask you questions such as "Have you always had cold hands?" "When did you start experiencing that?" "Have you been under stress lately?".

Medical History and Risk Factors

It is of great importance to give your doctor as many details about your health as possible:

-        Your usual state of health. Be sure to discuss any changes that you may have been experiencing.

-        The medical history of your family. This is especially important as your family medical history can be the cause of your hypothyroidism. Have any close family member suffered from thyroid dysfunction or any other autoimmune disease? Be sure to tell your doctor about it.

-        If you have had a neck radiation or thyroid surgery, your doctor must be immediately notified about it.

-        Make sure to give your doctor the list of medications you have been taking, even the most insignificant ones. Needless to say, if you have been taking heavy medicaments that may affect your thyroid function (see Medications), your doctor must know about it.

Physical Examination

Your doctor will most likely perform a physical examination and look for present physical signs of hypothyroidism, such as:

-        Slower reflexes

-        Swelling around the legs

- Swelling around the eyes

- Evidence of dry skin

- Slower heart rate

Blood Tests

The main purpose of the blood tests is to measure the T4 and the TSH levels. Usually, the typical person that has an underactive thyroid will have low levels of T4 and high levels of TSH. This means that his thyroid gland is not producing enough thyroid hormones and that the pituitary recognizes this as a problem, and immediately responds by releasing more TSH, in an attempt to force the thyroid to increase its production of hormones.

In the rate cases that we talked about earlier, where the problem is not in the thyroid but in the pituitary gland, there will be low levels of T4, but the TSH levels will also be low. In this case, the thyroid is responding to the hormone production request as it should, while the pituitary gland is not making enough TSH, which also results in inadequate amount of T4.

TSH TESTING

As we already said, the pituitary gland stimulates the production of the thyroid hormones T3 and T4 by releasing the TSH, so it is pretty obvious how the first line of testing is based on these levels. The TSH levels can be measured with a blood test.

The TSH levels are determined by ranges, and in milliunits per liter. The ranges below are according to the American Thyroid Association, however, keep in mind that they are not exactly set in stone. They can vary from person to person, from day to day, or even from lab to lab.

-        0.4 – normal

-        2.5 – at risk

-        4 – mild hypothyroidism

-        10 – hypothyroidism

These tests are very sensitive and in most cases, extremely accurate. With TSH testing, even the mildest cases can be successfully diagnosed.

T4 TESTING

The TSH testing may be accurate in diagnosing hypothyroidism, but that does not mean that just because that testing has come back normal your thyroid functions normally. You shouldn't rule out the possibility of hypothyroidism based on the normal TSH test. If you have many symptoms pointing towards an underactive thyroid, your doctor may suggest T4 testing.

The normal range for the levels of the T4 hormones is 5 to 13.5 micrograms per litter. If you have low T4 levels, that might be a solid indicator that you have hypothyroidism, even in the cases where the TSH test was normal.

ANTI-THYROID MICROSOMAL ANTIBODIES TESTING

The third test for checking for hypothyroidism is for anti-thyroid microsomal antibodies. These antibodies are produced by the immune system and can attack healthy thyroid cells. They are part of the body's autoimmune response, and if the blood test determines that they are present, that can be an indicator that there is some thyroid damage which can eventually lead to hypothyroidism. This is what characterizes the Hashimoto's thyroiditis.

Know that most primary doctors do not perform these kinds of tests so you may be referred to a specialist.

In a perfect case, your blood test result should be able to show the real situation with the thyroid. And the most individuals are diagnosed with hypothyroidism this way. However, there are millions of people struggling with this disorder undiagnosed. For those people, the solution is far more complex. Many blame the doctors saying that they use outdated lab ranges or that they fail to do full blood testing. Although we can agree that there are certain cases like that, that is surely not always the culprit. Your doctor can take into consideration every symptom and do every possible hypothyroidism test, and still fail to diagnose you. Why? Because in rare cases, these tests cannot show us the full picture.

The lab results, for instance, cannot test and show what actually happens with your thyroid hormones after they enter the cells in the body. Every bodily cell depends on these hormones, for sure, however, there is no test that can show us how well these cells actually utilize the thyroid hormones.

Each and every one is unique and has different requirements, just as not all cases of hypothyroidism are the same. We can neither predict how the patient will feel by examining the thyroid levels, and neither will those levels always be correct. The normal ranges are not that normal for some people. The goal shouldn't be about making the blood tests to be in the normal range, but for the person to feel better.

How Dangerous Is It?

The thyroid gland plays a hugely significant role to our hole. The hormones that it produces are important for keeping our metabolism balanced and they influence pretty much every single body function. They influence:

- Weight

- Body temperature

- Fertility

- Cardiovascular health

I am sure that you can all imagine the importance of the butterfly-shaped gland found in your neck. However, when the thyroid fails to produce and release the adequate amount of hormones, it disrupts the body's balance and causes the improper function of many body functions. But is this gland really that important and what happens if your underactive thyroid is left untreated?

Complications

Whether you have the mildest possible hypothyroidism or a full-blown condition, it is of utmost importance that you address this condition the right way immediately. If your hypothyroidism stays untreated it can quickly progress and cause a multitude of health problems.

The complications listed below all happen as a result of untreated hypothyroidism and can really take a toll on your overall health. Here is what you will be avoiding by seeking the right treatment for your hypothyroidism:

Goiter

In most cases, your thyroid doesn't just protest and willingly refuses to produce and release T3 and T4 hormones. Quite the contrary. The stimulation that comes from the pituitary gland surely touches your thyroid. The thyroid then tries to do its best to produce the required hormone levels, but for some reason, it fails. This exerting of the thyroid to keep up with the excessive stimulation demand and produce the adequate amount of hormones, in some cases, causes the thyroid to enlarge. This enlargement results with a bulge in your neck, which is known as goiter.

Birth Defects

Pregnant women with untreated hypothyroidism can pass many of the complications of this disorder on to their newborns. Babies that are born to women with hypothyroidism, in many cases, have much more birth defects than those born to healthy mothers. And I am not talking about insignificant complications; some serious mental and physical issues with the development can also occur. This is mainly because a healthy thyroid gland is fundamental for the proper development of the brain. Testing the thyroid function is part of the normal newborn screening. This includes blood tests to rule out any possible diseases.

Cardiovascular Problems

Even the mildest case of hypothermia can negatively affect your heart's health. This will result in slow and weekend pulse and abnormal heartbeats in the beginning, and if left untreated can progress to much more serious complications.

A thyroid that fails to produce enough hormones can increase the levels of your bad cholesterol and therefore contribute to the development of heart diseases, which is a clear indicator of how this condition increases your risk for strokes and heart attacks.

Hypothyroidism also contributes to pericardial effusion, which means that it will cause a buildup of fluid around your heart that will make it hard for your heart to pump blood efficiently. In fact, one study has shown that underactive thyroid can decrease the heart's ability to pump out blood by 30 – 50 percent. Fortunately, if this condition is addressed the right way, all of this can be easily prevented.

Infertility

Not having the adequate amount of hormones travel to our body cells can affect many functions, and ovulation, unfortunately, is one of them. This is probably the biggest negativity associated with hypothyroidism because in some cases, even if the hypothyroidism is treated, there is no guarantee that the hypothyroid woman can be fully fertile. That does not mean, however, that the women who struggle with this disorder cannot conceive.

Mental Health Issues

Having hypothyroidism that is not treated the right way can take a toll on your mental health as well. Since we mentioned depression in the symptoms earlier, you can imagine that this is a common complication associated with hypothyroidism. Mild forms of hypothyroidism can cause mild depression, however, as the hypothyroidism progresses so will the depression become more and more intense.

Also, there is evidence that proves that untreated hypothyroidism can result in a decrease in mental functioning over time.

Renal Complications

Your kidney is also affected by this vexing disorder. This also happens because the drop in thyroid hormones decreases the blood flow to the kidneys. This will leave the hypothyroid person unable to successfully absorb sodium by excreting water, which will result in low sodium levels.

Bleeding Issues

If your body produces insufficient thyroid hormones, the hypothyroidism can prevent the blood from clotting and may cause some heavy bleeding. Women will experience this in a form of very heavy menstrual cycles. Low production of blood cells along with heavy bleeding can easily result in anemia.

Nerve Damage

Underactive thyroid causes the buildup of fluids which will obviously lead to swelling. This will put an enormous pressure on your nerves and may damage, or even destroy them. This may result in peripheral neuropathy.

Of course, this type of nerve damage comes with an onset of symptoms. And while that mainly depends on the type of nerves that are affected, these are the most common signs of nerve damages:

- Muscle weakness

- Numbness

-      Burning

-      Tingling

-      Sensitivity to touch

Although not so common, hypothyroidism is also known to lead to carpal tunnel syndrome which causes pain, tingling, and numbness in the arm, wrist, and hand.

Breathing Problems

The weakness in the muscles caused by an underactive thyroid gland can also affect those muscles that help us breathe. When these muscles get weak people experience shortness of breath which most of the time leads to sleep apnea, or may even worsen it if the condition is already present.

Myxedema

We have mentioned this condition earlier when we talked about the symptoms of hypothyroidism, however, since it is life-threatening, I believe that it belongs in this list. Although myxedema is very rare because it is unlikely that you will not recognize the symptoms of such a progressed condition or that you will intentionally leave it untreated, however, in some rare cases, myxedema slows the metabolism to that point that the hypothyroid person falls into a coma. If you have extreme fatigue or a super high cold intolerance, seek emergency treatment immediately.

Treating the Underactive Thyroid

Hypothyroidism is a condition that is characterized by low thyroid hormones, so you have probably already guessed that the right treatment for this condition will be the replacement of the insufficient hormones. That therapy is known as thyroid hormone replacement therapy.

Thyroid Hormone Replacement Therapy

To better understand this therapy, you will need to have a solid knowledge of the interaction of the two thyroid hormones – T3 and T4.

T3 or triiodothyronine and T4 or tetraiodothyronine (also called thyroxine) control the metabolism of your body, and if your body lacks these hormones, the metabolism will obviously run slower. It is the rate of your metabolism that commands the way in which your body will function. The essential job of the T3 and T4 hormones is in the energy usage department.

But although they are produced by the same gland, these two hormones are not equally strong. T3 is more active than T4 and it has more strength. But while T3 may be stronger and more powerful, it is actually the T4 hormone that is taken during a standard thyroid hormone replacement therapy. You must wonder why that is. The reason behind that lies in the fact that most of the hormones T3 found in our body actually used to be T4s. It is the T4 hormones that come into contact with the cells in our bloodstream, and give each cell an iodine atom to interact with. Once the T4 become 1 iodine atom short, the hormone becomes T3.

Once this conversion of hormones occurs, the T3 immediately transports the metabolic message to the other cells in the body. It is a standard treatment to replace only the T4 hormones is for the purpose of allowing the body to perform the needed functions, which is converting T4s into T3s.

The Goal

If you have hypothyroidism, chances are you will be prescribed a thyroid hormone replacement therapy in order to compensate the insufficient amount of thyroid hormones released by this butterfly-shaped gland. In the majority of the cases, that is done by taking a T4 pill daily.

While this all seems like a standard and one-of-a-kind type of procedure, it is important for you to know that every therapy is different and tailored to the patient's unique needs. Every person absorbs the hormones in a different way and obviously needs a different amount to compensate, so you can expect to be prescribed an individualized therapy.

The goal of this therapy is to bring the thyroid stimulating hormone (TSH) levels to normal, so your doctor will everything to find the best treatment option for you.

Types of T4 Medications

There is not one but 6 synthetic T4 hormone supplements that are FDA approved.   Your doctor will most certainly prescribe you with one of these brands:

-        Synthroid

- Levoxyne

- Levo – T

- UNITHROID

- Novothyrox

- Levothyroxine Sodium

If you wonder which one of these supplements is the best, know that, despite the fact that they all replace the T4 hormones, they are not equal. So the question shouldn't be which one is the best, but which one is the best one for you. Obviously, only your doctor can give you that answer. However, the one supplement that is most commonly prescribed is Synthroid, because it delivers a prolonged and very steady dose of the T4 hormone.

All of the T4 medications listed above are bioequivalent, so there is not a significant difference in their composition. But again, they are not equal. Their composition may be the same, however, the way in which they are ingested is not. That is why the American Thyroid Association believes that once you begin taking one brand of T4 supplement, you should stick with it. Changing brands during this treatment is really not recommended (unless of course you experience some side effect or your doctor believes that you should benefit most from another brand), since by doing that you risk the return of the hypothyroidism symptoms. Another thing why this is not recommended is the fact that changing medications may also require a change in your dosage, which will also change the way you feel.

The Dosage

Finding the right dosage is as important as finding the right type of T4 supplement. The right one can keep the hypothyroidism from harming your health and interfering with your life, while the wrong one can make this condition even worse.

Finding the perfect dosage is indeed essential, however, keep in mind that the dosage you start with is not the one that you will keep. The dosage is usually determined by taking the body weight into consideration. If your treatment and hypothyroidism diet help you lose some weight, obviously, the dosage will not stay the same. The starting dosage is about 1.6 micrograms per every kilogram of weight. However, know that 1.6 micrograms is the full dose. If you perhaps have a part of your thyroid that functions properly, in that case, your doctor will prescribe a lower dose, as your gland will continue making some amount of T4 on its own.

Unfortunately, the thyroid hormone replacement therapy is a lifelong and permanent treatment. That being said, it is important to check yourself every year or so, to make sure that you are taking the right dosage.

The Symptoms of Over-Treatment

Even if your dose is moderate, there are still chances that your body will not get used to it, and you might experience some symptoms. It is important to be able to recognize if your body is not used with the prescribed dose so you can consult your doctor and adjust it accordingly. The symptoms of over-treatment include:

-        Sweating more than usual

-        Feeling hot

-        Muscle weakness

-        Weight loss

-        Having difficulty to fall asleep

-        Hand tremors and shaking

-        Mood swings

- Loss of concentration and memory loss

- Irregular menstrual cycle

T4 Supplements and Other Medications

Since you will be ingesting the T4 medications, it has to be absorbed into the bloodstream from your gastrointestinal tract. However, If there are other medications present in your GI tract, they can interfere with your ability to absorb the T4 hormone. And while not all medications will make slow down the absorptions, some may cause serious interference:

- Iron Supplements

- Aluminum Hydroxide

- Sucralfate

- Colestid and Cholestyramine

- Raloxifene

- Calcium Supplements

- Soy-Based Foods

If you need to take some of the medications from above, the safest way to do it is to take them at least 3 or 4 hours after or before you take your T4 supplement.

The effects of the thyroid hormone replacement therapy can be experienced approximately two weeks after starting to take the T4 supplements. If the T4 medication is taken at the right time and in the right dosage, it can successfully manage your underactive thyroid and not let the hypothyroidism interfere with your life.

The Right Kind of Diet

The food you consume, obviously, has a deep impact on your overall health. It can either pack you with the right kinds of nutrients or elevate your blood sugar and cholesterol levels. It is a well-known fact that we should be mindful about the kind of food we put on our dinner tables in order to be healthy. But when you already suffer from a vexing condition such as hypothyroidism, you should be extra careful with your diet, as its guidelines slightly change course when you have such a disorder to think about. But, before we start restocking your kitchen with food that will help you boost the release of thyroid hormones, there are two huge misconceptions that I believe are extremely important to be clarified first:

#1: Your Hypothyroidism Diet Is Enough to Treat Your Underactive Thyroid

If only it were that simple. The truth is, there is no such diet that can cure your hypothyroidism. You may be the most disciplined dieter and never have a bite of something that will not benefit your thyroid gland, but in the end, you still will not be able to prevent your lack of thyroid hormones from interfering with your life. Why? Because this diet cannot work alone. The hypothyroidism diet cannot treat this condition on its own unless it is combined with the regular consumption of the right dosage of T4 medication. So why even bother, you may wonder. Why even try to sacrifice your sugar-loaded desserts and juicy junk food if you cannot treat your disorder that way. Because your T4 medication cannot work on its own either. The only way in which you can live a normal and healthy life is if this diet joins forces with the supplements that your doctor have prescribed. Because if you continue with your unbalanced diet and be nutrient deficient, the T4 supplement will not effectively treat the hypothyroidism.

#2: Desiccated Thyroid Is Not the Solution

If you were thinking about finding an alternative medicine that can completely replace your conventional T4 supplement, let me break it to you – there isn't one. There are those alternative medicine advocates that swear by the effectiveness of the consumption of desiccated thyroid, however, that has not been scientifically proven.

Desiccated thyroid, which is basically a ground-up pork thyroid, actually contains a mixture of both T3 and T4 hormones, which hasn't proven to be as effective as the artificial T4 medications.

Sure, I am all about organic and 100 % natural when it comes to our health, but when you are dealing with a condition that can threaten your life if not treated the right way, I say we stick to what has already been proven and stop experimenting with our lives.

Now that we have these misconceptions out of our way, we can proceed towards finding the right dietary balance that can help us get our thyroid hormone levels in check.

Foods to Eat

If you have already been diagnosed with hypothyroidism then you have also been advised to follow a strict hypothyroidism diet. And while we said how the diet itself cannot help you treat your underactive thyroid permanently, a modification and healthifying of your diet is indeed an essential step towards giving your low thyroid hormones a boost.

Just like with any other type of diet, there are some foods that are beneficial, and some foods that may hurt your condition. Be sure to pack your kitchen with this thyroid-friendly ingredients:

Fish. Providing you with omega-3 fatty acids that are crucial for the proper thyroid function and the right hormonal balance, fish should be a regular guest on your dinner table. If you balance the intake of omega-3 and omega-6 fatty acids, your hypothyroidism diet can actually help you fight off inflammation and provide a good support for your healthy neurological function.

Wild caught fish such as Pacific sardines or Atlantic mackerel are the best sources of omega-3s. But that doesn't mean that canned tuna is no good for you. Canned tuna, actually, is a pretty decent source of iodine, which is essential for your hypothyroidism diet. Only 3 ounces of canned tuna will provide you with 17 micrograms of iodine, which is 11 percent of the recommended daily intake. 3 ounces of cod, on the other hand, will pack you with 66 % of the recommended daily intake of iodine, which is 99 micrograms. Pretty amazing, right?

Shellfish. Shellfish is also a great source of iodine and a healthy addition to your hypothyroidism diet. Although it is pretty hard to determine exactly how much iodine foods that are not fortified with it contain (since iodine is not listed on the product unless it is fortified), we can believe the general rule that the shrimp, crab, and lobster are great sources of iodine. In fact, 3 ounces of shrimp contains more than 20 percent of the recommended daily value. Besides, shellfish is also packed with zinc, which is also beneficial.

Coconut Oil. This ingredient really is a staple of this hypothyroidism diet. Providing beneficial fatty acids in the form of lauric, capric, and caprylic acid, coconut oil supports the metabolism by fighting fatigue and increasing one's energy. Packed with antioxidant, antimicrobial, and antibacterial properties that fight inflammation and supports digestion, coconut oil will especially be helpful for treating autoimmune diseases, Hashimoto's thyroiditis included.

Seaweed. Seaweed is actually chockfull of beneficial iodine content, which can prevent those deficiencies that disrupt the normal thyroid function. It is highly recommended that you enjoy seaweed once a week for best results. Try nori, wakame, dulse, kombu, and kelp. Use them in soup, salads, sushi, risotto, in fish cakes, or however you like. I only suggest it once a week because seaweed is really high in iodine and since we said that too much iodine can also be harmful, once a week is the perfect dose.

Foods Rich in Probiotic. It is a common fact that probiotic supports the microflora bacteria and therefore is essential for balancing your gut. Since we said how in many cases the leaky gut is actually to blame for the hypothyroidism, you can only assume that probiotic-rich food can destroy inflammation, autoimmune disorders, and with that support the production of the thyroid hormones. Great choices of foods that are rich in probiotic include:

- Kefir

- Organic Yogurt, especially goat's milk yogurt

- Kombucha

- Kimchi

- Natto

- Sauerkraut

- Other fermented veggies

Sprouted Seeds. Seeds such as hemp, chia, and flax seeds provide with a beneficial type of omega-3 fatty acids called ALA. This is crucial for the normal thyroid function and therefore will be extremely beneficial for your health if incorporated into your hypothyroidism diet.

Not only sprouted seeds, but all healthy fats should also be a part of your hypothyroidism diet because they will not only boost the hormonal production but also lower the blood sugar and help you lose or maintain weight.

Grains. All grains that do not contain gluten is not only welcome but also necessary to be incorporated into your Hypothyroidism diet. Not only they can be used to create delicious recipes with, but they are packed with powerful nutrients that can stimulate your thyroid gland to be better at doing its job. Here are the best choices for your thyroid:

- Quinoa

- Buckwheat

- Brown Rice

- Amaranth

- Wild Rice

Brazil Nuts. Speaking of healthy fats, nuts, in general, are really healthy and welcome in your diet, and especially brazil nuts. Brazil nuts stand out from the others in this food category, simply because they are rich in selenium – a helpful nutrient that is successful in regulating the thyroid function, thanks to the great job it does at converting the T4 thyroid hormone to T3. One French study conducted on women has shown that those who consume more selenium have lower chances for developing goiters and damage of the thyroid tissue. Plus, it is super helpful for those who already have Hashimoto's thyroiditis, because this nutrient can stave off the permanent damage that has already been made.

However, as beneficial as Brazil nuts are, that doesn't mean that it is safe for you to munch on them all the time. Keep in mind that your body needs only a small amount of selenium in order to nudge the thyroid to function the right way.

Chicken and Beef. If you are a meat lover, here are some good news – you can enjoy chicken and beef safely on the hypothyroidism diet. Although other types of meat such as pork aren't exactly forbidden, know that they are also not especially recommended, so please be moderate if you cannot resist a pork chop once in a while.

Chicken and beef should be an essential part of your diet because they will pack you with adequate amounts of zinc. And since zinc is great for churning out the thyroid hormones, lean cuts of meat are therefore welcome to your hypothyroidism diet. Another thing why they will do wonders for your thyroid is the fact that they are high in tyrosine – an amino acid that joins forces with iodine and supports the balanced functioning of the thyroid.

Please note that the meat you are buying should be 100 % organic and grass-fed only. Commercially raised animals are often fed antibiotics which can be pretty troublesome for your thyroid gland.

Eggs. Do you know that a single large egg contains approximately 16 % of the needed daily value of iodine, and 20 % of the recommended daily intake of selenium, which makes eggs super thyroid friendly. Unless your doctor has suggested otherwise, eggs should be a part of your breakfast meals.

Your thyroid craves an adequate protein consumptions, and enriching your diet with breakfast eggs is one of the best way to ensure that the needed protein intake is received.

Just like meat, your eggs should also be organic and free range. The antibiotics that commercial chickens are packed with pollutes the egg too, so make sure that you will not disrupt your thyroid function by buying them.

Foods that are High in Fiber. You know how fiber supports digestion? Well, since those who have hypothyroidism are known to have digestive problems, fiber is very much welcome in your hypothyroidism diet. Plus, fiber can balance your blood sugar levels, help you with your weight loss/maintenance goal, and support heart health. Include more berries, fresh veggies, beans, lentils, and seeds, in your diet.

Beans are extremely important for your Hypothyroidism, not only because they are packed with fiber, but also because of their rich iodine content. Make sure to include a variety of beans in your diet for best results:

- Black Beans

- Navy Beans

- Red Kidney Beans

- Azuki Beans

- Lima Beans

- Pinto Beans

- Mung Beans

Fruits and Veggies. High in minerals, vitamins, and rich in antioxidants, fruits and veggies are fundamental for battling inflammation and destroying the free-radical damage. Since they are so nutrient dense, fresh fruits and veggies should make up a huge portion of your diet.

Vegetables – Although there is no healthy diet without an abundance of fresh veggies, here are the best choices that will support a proper thyroid function:

Artichokes – When it comes to the thyroid, artichokes are a real superfood. Packed with the most powerful antioxidant and cleansing properties, adding artichokes to your hypothyroid plate will lead to a total liver cleanse. Being great at detoxifying the liver, artichokes can make a real difference on your journey to healing the thyroid.

Since people with Hashimoto's are known to have reduced detoxifying abilities, and your liver, well, is the primary detoxification organ, you can do the math and see how a simple habit of adding a few artichoke hearts to your meal can be so successful in kicking the thyroid to function properly.

Potatoes – Potatoes are a powerful source of tyrosine which your underactive thyroid needs in order to become better at doing its job.

Other great choices of veggies include:

- Beets

- Carrots

- Cucumber

- Mushrooms

- Peppers

- Pumpkin

- Tomatoes

- Squash

- Zucchini

- Celery

Fruits – Although we know how we should be somewhat more mindful about eating fruits because of their fructose content, most of them are packed with a great deal of nutrients that can help you treat your condition.

Avocados – Although this one probably goes without saying, since there is no diet in the world that does not encourage the consumption of avocados, they are especially great for your thyroid because of the fact that they are packed with tyrosine. And since having an underactive thyroid means being short in this beneficial amino acid, you can see the importance of the avocado consumption.

Cranberries – All berries in genera will bring benefits to your thyroid, however, cranberries are the ones that are packed with iodine the most. A single cup of cranberries contain incredible 400 mcg of iodine, so you can see how great would be if you added a handful of this fruit here and there.

Other great fruit choices include:

- Apples

- Kiwi

- Pineapple

- Citrud Fruit, Grapefruits especially

- Apricots

- Bananas

- Cherries

- Grapes

Bone Broth. Although chicken and beef broth are also beneficial since they contain amino acids that can help you boost the thyroid function, bone broth is especially recommended. Bone broth contains a high amount of minerals that can help you nourish the digestive tract, overcome food sensitivities, fight fatigue, increase the energy levels, and lower the pain in the muscles, all of which are associated with hypothyroidism.

Healthy Oils. Forget about vegetable and refined oils and pack your diet with the healthy choices below, because they are all known to hold a pretty powerful stimulating effect over your butterfly-shaped gland:

- Olive Oil

- Coconut Oil

- Butter

Herbs. Herbs are famous for being detoxifying powerhouses, but the ones you will see below will especially trigger your thyroid to produce more of the T3 and T4 hormones. They will not only purge the toxins such as mercury from your body, but they will also rasie your whole metabolism as well. Be sure to include:

- Garlic

- Cilantro

- Black Pepper

- Turmeric

- Parsley

- Peppermint

- Rosemary

- Ginger

- Cinnamon

Foods to Avoid

Since almost 90 percent of the hypothyroid cases are a result of autoimmune diseases, it is clear that a person's diet can be highly linked to this condition. Changing and modifying your diet can be the best weapon that will help you stop hypothyroidism from harming your health.

If you haven't done it already, this is the perfect time to get everything out of the fridge, pantry, and shelves, and do a full kitchen makeover. The foods listed below can interfere with your thyroid goals, so make sure to get rid of them.

Goitrogen Foods. There has been a huge misconception wrapped around the cruciferous vegetables. Are they good or dangerous for hypothyroidism? Should you steam them or at raw? Well, this is a little bit murky, to be honest. Cruciferous vegetables such as broccoli, kale, Brussel sprouts, cauliflower, cabbage, and soy, actually contain goitrogens – which are molecules that can damage the thyroid peroxidase. So, you should steer clear from them at any cost, right? Not so much. They are fine to eat in moderation, but after being steamed for 30 minutes. You should never eat raw cruciferous veggies. If you eat normal serving sizes from time to time, it is really highly unlikely that these veggies can hurt your thyroid in some way.

Gluten. Ah, the good old gluten controversy. To go or not to go against the grains? Well, if you have hypothyroidism and want to treat it, then you should definitely avoid consuming grains that contain gluten. Most people who have thyroid dysfunctions are either pretty sensitive to gluten or they have celiac disease – which is an autoimmune disease that results in becoming allergic to gluten. What, rye and barley, and every product that is made from these ingredients should be avoided.

Many packaged foods seem to contain gluten these days, so be sure to check the label ingredients before buying a new product.

Sugar. Probably the most obvious hazard to any diet and disease – is sugar. It can seriously disrupt the normal metabolic balance that can lead to a number of other health issues. People suffering from hypothyroidism have troubles shedding pounds as it is, and they really don't need sugar to make this process even harder than it already is. Besides, sugar can contribute to hormonal imbalances, mood swings, fatigue, and depression, which are also ways in which this sweet danger can hurt your thyroid.

Conventional Dairy. Just like sugar, conventional dairy can also be quite problematic for your thyroid, as it can support inflammation and raise its responses. Cow milk's products that are not organic and are pasteurized should be avoided at any cost. Instead, try consuming organic A2 cow's milk or goat's milk.

Refined Flour Products. Although we said how gluten should be avoided, and that obviously includes wheat and all of wheat's products, it is important to mention that any type of refined carbohydrates should also be avoided. Refined flour products can impact your hormone levels negatively and support hypothyroidism. If it is possible, it is recommended to remove most grains from your diet. If you have to, choose 100 organic and gluten-free grains such as quinoa or buckwheat.

Supplements for Your Hypothyroidism Diet

Yes, the hypothyroidism diet and your T4 medication together can really help you live a long and normal life and never experience any of the unwanted symptoms that may occur as a result of having an underactive thyroid. However, that does not mean that you will never be deficient of a nutrient or that you will consume all of the important vitamins and minerals through your diet only.

In case you have to incorporate a supplement or two into your diet, here are the natural supplements that have proven to be the most successful remedies for those struggling with hypothyroidism:

Iodine. Although we have already mentioned this nutrient a couple of times, emphasizing the huge part that it plays in restoring the thyroid health and balancing the hormones, sometimes consuming iodine from your food is not enough to provide you with the sufficient benefits. Many studies have proven that even the tiniest amounts of supplemental iodine can be extremely helpful for your condition. If you choose to take anywhere from 150 to 300 micrograms of iodine daily, you can soon experience significant changes in your T3 and T4 hormones.

However, you need to keep in mind that iodine supplement is not recommended for those who struggle with Hashimoto's thyroiditis, since getting too much iodine may have a counter effect and help your body develop an overactive thyroid and welcome hyperthyroidism instead.

And while it is super rare to exceed the upper daily limit of iodine, sometimes that can be done if you eat too much seaweed or take this supplement.

Selenium. Do you know that your thyroid gland is the only organ in your body that has such a high content of selenium? That is because selenium is especially important in the production of thyroid hormones, as well as for reducing the effects caused by autoimmune diseases. That being said, you can imagine how important selenium is for your hypothyroidism diet. And while there are certain types of food that may provide you with a substantial selenium content such as brazil nuts, beef, chicken, yellowfin tuna, sardines, halibut, etc., that usually isn't enough and selenium supplement is needed.

Selenium supplement is especially beneficial for those suffering from Hashimoto's thyroiditis, as well as pregnant women because for them, it can decrease the level of the antibody levels that are not thyroid friendly, as well as improve the thyroid's structure. Because it is so effective in balancing the hormone levels, 200 micrograms of selenium supplement are welcome daily.

Ashwagandha. This is an adaptogen herb that is in charge of keeping the hormones balanced and helping the body respond to stress the right way. Ashwagandha is super useful because it can not only balance the T4 levels, but also lower the cortisol. Studies have shown that taking ashwagandha supplement for 8 weeks results in an increase in the levels of the thyroxine hormone, which in turn lowers the intensity of the hypothyroidism. The recommended dosage is 500 milligrams a day.

Similar adaptogens are holy basil, licorice root, ginseng, and Rhodiola, and they will have a very similar effect.

L-Tyrosine. Used in the synthesis of the hormones produced by the thyroid, this amino acid is originally produced with the tyrosine iodination. This supplement is extremely beneficial in improving sleep disorders, reducing fatigue, and increasing alertness. The reason why this amino acid is beneficial for your thyroid function is that it is a part of the natural 'feel good' hormones such as melatonin, norepinephrine, and dopamine. The recommended dosage is 500 milligrams, twice a day.

Fish Oil. Omega-3 fatty acids are extremely important not only for your overall health but for treating hypothyroidism and improving the T3 and T4 production, as well. The main source of these beneficial fatty acids is of course fish. However, if you do not eat fish, or you do not consume the required amount of omega-3 fatty acids on daily basis, then taking a fish oil supplement is probably the best choice. The recommended dosage is 1000 milligrams daily.

Probiotic Supplement. Probiotics are very important in retrieving the gut balance because they support the nutrient absorption while lowering the inflammation at the same time. Probiotics also help with appetite control and weight maintenance, so they are pretty important for improving the thyroid function, as well. If you experience gut problems, as many hypothyroid people do, do not hesitate to go to the pharmacy and buy a probiotic supplement. It can only do you good.

Vitamin B-Complex. Playing a hugely important part in balancing the hormones and the proper neurological function, vitamin B12 and thiamine are essential in the hypothyroidism diet. There are studies that have shown that consuming thiamine supplements regularly can help you defeat autoimmune diseases. In fact, one clinical study where patients with Hashimoto's disease were given 600 milligrams of thiamine supplement per day has shown that thiamine helps with fatigue regression after only a few hours.

Vitamin B12 is also crucial for combating fatigue because it provides the central nervous system with a number of benefits such as maintaining and protecting the health of the nerve cells.

Simple Dietary and Lifestyle Tips

It is not all about what you eat, but how you eat it as well. We have covered the foods that should and shouldn't be in your diet, now all that is left is to add some simple, but extremely important dietary tips that will ensure that you stay on the right track of your hypothyroidism diet and moving in the right direction towards boosting the production and release of the thyroid hormones.

Besides dietary tips, this chapter will also teach you what lifestyle changes you need to make, in order to give your maximum support to the thyroid and support its proper function.

Here is what you need to have in mind while fighting hypothyroidism:

- Make sure to drink clean water. The water you drink must be filtered in order to help you with hydration and prevent moodiness and fatigue. Tap water contains fluorine which has the power to prevent the absorption of iodine, so it should be avoided. Aim to drink at least 8 ounces of clean water every two hours.

- Find out if you are food intolerant. Make sure that before you start this diet you exclude every food that you are sensitive to or that it burdens your digestive tract. The hypothyroidism diet is all about feeling good and bringing balance to your body, so if any type of food brings you discomfort, make sure to avoid eating it.

- Opt for buying only 100 % natural and organic products, and make sure to always read the labels when buying products from different manufacturer (even if the food is the same), as the ingredients vary from one manufacturer to another, and just because the brand you used to buy didn't include gluten, it doesn't mean that other brands don't either.

- Limit your alcohol intake. I am not saying that you should abstain from having a drink completely, however, rethink the refill. One glass of wine here and there will not hurt you – in fact, it has been known to be quite healthy – however having three or four will definitely have a counter effect and may disrupt the balance of the thyroid hormones.

- Do a liver detox from time to time, as this is where the T4 into T3 hormone conversion actually happens. This can be done by taking turmeric supplement, eating more potassium, ditch coffee, and drinking raw veggie juices. Some beef liver may also be good for cleansing the liver.

- Avoid drinking store-bought smoothies or fruit juices, even if they say that they are 100 percent natural since in the majority of the cases they are packed with sugar. You may up your vitamin intake by drinking them, however, consuming sugar can disrupt the hormonal balance in your body.

- Stay clear of junk food and empty calories. Make sure to eat only nutritious food and do not cheat. Your thyroid will know it.

- Always eat in a relaxed environment. Avoid eating while pushing the deadline in your office in front of your computer and over a bunch of documents. No matter how busy you are, always try to set some time aside for eating. This will give your body the best opportunity to digest the food the right way, and absorb its nutrients. This way you will avoid spiking up your stress levels and hurting your thyroid function even more.

- Quit smoking. It is a common knowledge that cigarette smoke releases number of toxins. One of these toxins is thiocyanate, which is especially dangerous for your thyroid as it can support its dysfunction.

People who smoke are also susceptible to developing thyroid eye complications as a result of the Grave's disease. Needless to say, cigarettes are bad for your overall health.

- Buy only fluoride-free toothpaste. Fluoride is actually used for lowering the production of thyroid hormones, usually for those that suffer from hyperthyroidism, and can seriously disrupt the hormonal balance that you try to achieve through the proper diet and medications.

-      Exercise. Although this hypothyroidism diet is definitely the cornerstone of the treatment of your underactive thyroid gland, you cannot possibly achieve the desired results if you are leading a sedentary lifestyle. Remember how we said that inactivity is one of the causes for this awful condition? Well, guess what? Once you develop it, staying inactive can only make things worse. It is of great importance that you exercise on regular basis to support the balanced release of hormones. If your days are hectic and super busy and you cannot find time for exercise, that doesn't excuse you for not being active.

Getting up 20 minutes earlier to go for a quick jog will not affect your beauty sleep, and so won't getting off the bus two stops earlier and walking to work, taking the stairs instead of the elevator, doing a few crunches, push-ups after eating instead of hugging the couch, etc. Being active doesn't necessarily mean spending hours in the gym.

21-Day Hypothyroidism Diet Meal Plan

If the hypothyroidism diet seems overwhelming to you and you have no idea how to create a healthy meal plan and cook thyroid-friendly meals with the allowed ingredients only, do not worry. This chapter will help you gain a better understanding of all of the meal possibilities that you can enjoy while treating your thyroid.

Providing you with a full and carefully created a 21-day meal plan that will keep your thyroid hormones in check, as well as your weight, blood sugar, cholesterol levels, and your overall health balanced, with this meal plan you can safely start the hypothyroidism diet and still get to enjoy delicious food.

Day 1:

Breakfast:

2 hardboiled Eggs
1 Avocado
½ Tomato
1 Apple
½ cup Yogurt

Snack 1:

A handful of Pine Nuts

Lunch:

1 cup of Chicken Noodles Soup made with gluten-free noodles
1 cup Spinach and Lettuce salad
A handful of Berries

Snack 2:

1 Muffin made with Coconut or Almond Flour

Dinner:

4-ounces Salmon fillet
4 Asparagus Spears, steamed
1 Carrot, steamed
1 Potato, boiled
½ cup of Fruit Juice

Day 2:

Breakfast:

1 slice of gluten-free Toast
1 tbsp of organic Cottage Cheese
1 poached Egg
½ cup sliced Veggies

Snack 1:

1 Banana

Lunch:

1 can Tuna
½ small Cucumber
½ Tomato
1 cup Lettuce
2 tbsp Corn

Snack 2:

½ cup Kefir
1 piece of Fruit

Dinner:

4-ounce Beef Steak
½ cup mashed Potatoes
1/2 Bell Pepper
3 ounces grilled Mushrooms
½ cup of Fruit Juice

Day 3:

Breakfast:

¾ cup cooked Quinoa
½ cup sliced Fruit
½ cup Organic Milk

Snack 1:

1 Pear
A handful of Nuts

Lunch:

2 slices of gluten-free Bread
3 ounces of cooked and shredded Chicken
1 Lettuce Leaf
2 Tomato Slices
1 tsp Mustard

Snack 2:

1 cup Yogurt
1 tbsp Flax Seeds
2 tbsp mashed Berries

Dinner:

1 cup of Beef Stew
1 cup of Salad by choice
½ cup Fruit Juice

Day 4:

Breakfast:

1 Hard-Boiled Egg
1 slice of Gluten-Free Bread, toasted
1 tbsp Cream Cheese
½ cup Kefir
4 Cherry Tomatoes

Snack 1:

1 cup Apple Cinnamon Chips (baked apple slices sprinkled with cinnamon)

Lunch:

1 cup Red Lentil Soup
1 cup mixed Green Salad
½ cup Green Grapes

Snack 2:

2 tbsp Bean Dip
3 Baby Carrots
½ Cucumber, cut into strips
1 Peach

Dinner:

1 Gluten-Free Hamburger Bun
4 ounces pulled lean Beef
1 ½ tbsp Sauerkraut
2 Lettuce Leaves
4 Tomato Slices
1 tbsp Sauce by choice (made with allowed ingredients)
A handful of Berries

Day 5:

Breakfast:

1 cup of Chia Pudding

Snack 1:

1 cup of Grapes
4 Brazil Nuts

Lunch:

1 cup of Creamy Vegetable Soup
2 tbsp gluten-free croutons
1 tbsp Sunflower Seeds
1 Apple

Snack 2:

4 sugar-free and gluten-free Biscuits
½ cup of Organic Milk

Dinner:

¾ cup of cooked Rice
4 Jumbo Shrimp, grilled
1 Carrot, cooked
1 sheet of Nori
Sugar-Free Frozen Yogurt

Day 6:

Breakfast:

½ Avocado
1 poached Egg
1 slice of gluten-free Bread, toasted
1 tbsp of organic Cream Cheese

Snack 1:

1 cup of Popcorn
1 glass of Fruit Juice

Lunch:

2 Crab Cakes
½ cup cooked Rice
1 cup Salad
1 Kiwi

Snack 2:

1 cup of Yogurt
1 tbsp chopped Nuts
1 tbsp Seeds by choice
A handful of Berries

Dinner:

½ cup cooked Beans
4-ounce cooked Chicken
4 Cherry Tomatoes
2 Asparagus Spears
½ cup Red Grapes

Day 7:

Breakfast:

2 slices of gluten-free Bread, toasted
1 tbsp Coconut Oil
2 tbsp mashed Fruit by choice
1 cup of Organic Milk

Snack 1:

½ cup of Melon Chunks
A handful of Walnuts

Lunch:

1 cup of Pumpkin Soup
2 tbsp Pumpkin Seeds
1 tbsp Organic Sour Cream
2 tbsp gluten-free Croutons
½ Apple

Snack 2:

1 cup of baked Potato Chips seasoned with Turmeric
1 cup of Fruit Juice

Dinner:

1 cup Spaghetti Squash
¼ cup of Bolognese Sauce
A handful of Berries

Day 8:

Breakfast:

1 cup of Smoothie made with 1 Kiwi, 2 tbsp Chia Seeds, ½ cup Yogurt, A handful of Spinach, A handful of Almonds, Coconut Water, ¼ Avocado

Snack 1:

1 cup Watermelon Chunks
4 Brazil Nuts

Lunch:

Pesto Pasta made with Zoodles (Zucchini noodles)
½ cup Vegetable Juice

Snack 2:

2 Chocolate Chip Cookies (gluten-free, sugar-free, and with dark chocolate)
½ cup Organic Milk

Dinner:

1 cup of Fish Stew
1 slice of gluten-free Bread
1 glass of Lemonade

Day 9:

Breakfast:

Spinach and Onion omelet made with 2 Eggs
1 slice of gluten-free Bread
½ cup of Orange Juice

Snack 1:

1 Corn on the Cob

Lunch:

2 Lobster Rolls
½ cup of Pineapple Chunks

Snack 2:

1 cup of Kefir
1 tbsp chopped Nuts
1 tbsp Seeds
1/3 cup chopped Fruits

Dinner:

4 ounces Pot Roast
½ Sweet Potato, baked
1 Carrot, baked
1 cup of Salad made with Cucumbers, Lettuce, Tomatoes, and Red Onion

Day 10:

Breakfast:

2 gluten-free Pancakes
1/3 cup of chopped Fruits
½ cup Yogurt

Snack 1:

2 sugar-free and gluten-free Biscuits
½ Banana
2 Brazil Nuts

Lunch:

4 medium Shrimp, cooked
1 cup of Squash spaghetti
2 tbsp of Sauce made with allowed ingredients
½ Apple

Snack 2:

½ cup Veggie Medley, fermented
2 Rice Cakes

Dinner:

Hamburger made with 1 gluten-free Bun, 3-ounce Beef Pattie, 1 Lettuce Leaf, A couple of Onion Rings, 1 sliced Pickle, 2 Tomato Slices
½ cup Fruit Juice, optional

Day 11:

Breakfast:

1 serving (about 1 cup) of Sweet Potato Hash made with Eggs, Parsley, Mint, and Organic Feta Cheese
½ cup Orange Juice

Snack 1:

1 cup of Cucumber and Carrot Sticks
1 tbsp Hummus
1 tbsp Organic Cottage Cheese

Lunch:

1 cup of White Bean Soup
1 slice of gluten-free Bread
1/3 cup Sauerkraut

Snack 2:

1 cup of Cinnamon Rice Pudding made with Organic Milk

Dinner:

1 Chicken Drumstick, roasted
¼ Eggplant, roasted
¼ Zucchini, roasted
1 Carrot, roasted
1 Potato, roasted

Day 12:

Breakfast:

1 gluten-free Bagel
2 ounces Smoked Salmon
1 tbsp organic Cream Cheese
½ cup of Orange Juice

Snack 1:

1 cup of roasted and spiced Chickpeas

Lunch:

Quinoa Fruit Salad made with ¾ cup cooked Quinoa, 2 tbsp Coconut Flakes, 2 tbsp shaved Almonds, ½ cup of chopped fruit

Snack 2:

1 gluten-free and sugar-free Vanilla Muffin
½ cup Organic Milk

Dinner:

1 cup of Bean Chili made with allowed ingredients
½ cup Sauerkraut
A handful of Berries

Day 13:

Breakfast:

1 serving of Veggie Quiche made with Eggs, allowed Veggies, and organic Ricotta Cheese
1 Apple

Snack 1:

Smoothie made with 1 Banana, 1 tbsp sugar-free Cashew Butter, ½ cup of Milk, 1 tbsp Hemp Seeds, ¼ Avocado, water as needed

Lunch:

1 cup Rice Noodles
3 ounces flaked Fish by choice
¼ Cucumber
½ Bell Pepper

Snack 2:

1 cup of Popcorn
½ cup of Cranberry Juice

Dinner:

1 cup of Zucchini Noodles
2 ounces sautéed Mushrooms
2 tbsp Pasta sauce made with allowed ingredients
3 ounces cooked and shredded Turkey meat
½ cup frozen Red Grapes

Day 14:

Breakfast:

¼ Avocado, sliced
1 piece of gluten-free Bread, toasted
1 poached or hardboiled Egg
4 Cherry Tomatoes
¼ cup Yogurt

Snack 1:

1 serving of gluten-free and sugar-free Peach crumble

Lunch:

½ cup of cooked Rice with 1 sheet of Kelp
3 ounces sautéed Mushrooms
1 tbsp White Pasta Sauce made with allowed ingredients
1 Apricot

Snack 1:

1 Celery Stick
1 Carrot
¼ Cucumber
2 tbsp Hummus
½ cup Fruit Juice

Dinner:

4 ounces pulled roasted and pulled Beef
½ Potato, baked
½ Turnip, baked
1 cup of Salad by choice

Day 15:

Breakfast:

½ cup cooked Buckwheat
½ cup Coconut Milk
1 tbsp chopped Nuts
½ Banana

Snack 1:

½ cup Fruit Chunks by choice
2 Brazil Nuts

Lunch:

1 cup Onion Soup
2 tbsp gluten-free Croutons
1 cup Cucumber, Basil, Yogurt, and Parsley Salad

Snack 2:

1 cup Zucchini Chips

Dinner:

1 Salmon Fillet, baked
1 Potato, boiled
A handful of Spinach, steamed
¼ tbsp frozen Blueberries

Day 16:

Breakfast:

2 scrambled Eggs
1 ounce Organic Mozzarella Cheese
1 slice of gluten-free Bread, toasted
½ cup Orange Juice

Snack 1:

½ cup Pomegranate Molasses
A handful of mixed Nuts

Lunch:

1 canned Tuna
¼ cup Yogurt
A handful of chopped Parsley
½ Cucumber
1 Peach

Snack 2:

1 cup Popcorn
1 glass of Vegetable Juice

Dinner:

1 cup of Vegetable Stew
1 slice of gluten-free Bread
A handful of Berries

Day 17:

Breakfast:

1 Breakfast Smoothie Bowl made with ½ Avocado, ½ Banana, ½ Apple, 2 tbsp chopped Nuts, 1 tbsp Chia Seeds, 1 tbsp Flaxseeds, and Coconut Milk, as needed

Snack 1:

2 Sweet Potato Fritters
½ cup Yogurt

Lunch:

Risotto made with 1/3 cup Crab Meat, 2/3 cup Rice, 2 ounces sauteed Mushrooms, 1 tbsp of favorite Sauce with allowed ingredients
1 Orange

Snack 2:

2 Rice Cakes
2 Brazil Nuts
1 small Apricot

Dinner:

1 Corn Tortilla
2 tbsp Black Beans
1 tbsp Cannellini Beans
1 diced Tomato
1 tbsp sauce by choice, made with allowed ingredients
½ Bell Pepper
½ cup Fruit Juice

Day 18:

Breakfast:

2 Crepes made with Almond or Coconut Flour stuffed with mashed Berries, chopped Nuts, coconut flakes, and some yogurt

Snack 1:

2 Baby Carrots
1 Bell Pepper
2 tbsp Hummus

Lunch:

1 cup of Lentil Soup
1 cup of salad by choice

Snack 2:

1 Banana
4 Brazil Nuts

Dinner:

5 ounces cooked and shredded favorite Meat
1 cup Salad by choice
1 baked Potato
½ cup Pomegranate Molasses

Day 19:

Breakfast:

2 Hardboiled Eggs
1 slice of gluten-free Bread, toasted
1 ounce Organic Mozzarella
4 Cherry Tomatoes

Snack 1:

½ cup Watermelon Chunks
A handful of Walnuts

Lunch:

3 ounces flaked Fish
¾ cup Rice Noodles
½ cup Arugula with Olive Oil and Balsamic Vinegar (you can also add some nuts)

Snack 2:

½ cup Yogurt
1 tbsp Hemp Seeds
A handful of Berries

Dinner:

Sloppy Joes made with 1 gluten-free Bun, 4 ounces of cooked and shredded Beef, 1 tbsp of allowed Sauce, and 2 tbsp Sauerkraut

Day 20:

Breakfast:

2 Pancakes
¼ cup Yogurt
2 tbsp Blueberries
2 Strawberries
¼ Banana

Snack 1:

3 Gluten-Free Crackers
1 Peach

Lunch:

1 serving of Potato Salad made with 1 Large Potato, allowed raw greens,
mustard, yogurt, Red Onion, Parsley, Mint
½ cup of Fruit Juice

Snack 2:

1 cup of baked Potato Chips

Dinner:

4 large Shrimp
¾ cooked Rice
½ cup chopped and steamed Veggies

Day 21:

Breakfast:

1 poached Egg
½ Avocado, sliced
1 slice of gluten-free Bread, toasted
A handful of Spinach

Snack 1:

1 Banana
A handful of Nuts

Lunch:

3 ounces cooked and shredded Chicken
1 cup of clear Veggie Soup
½ cup Rice Noodles
1 Peach

Snack 2:

2 gluten-free and sugar-free Biscuits
½ cup Organic Milk

Dinner:

4 ounces flaked Fish
1 sheet of Nori
2/3 cup cooked Rice
3 ounces sautéed Mushrooms with some Onions
1 cup Salad by Choice
½ cup frozen Berries

Essential Oils Remedies for Your Hypothyroidism

Essential oils are known to leave a magical touch on pretty much everything that they are used for, and your thyroid function is not an exception. I am not saying that rubbing oils can actually cure this condition, however, if you want to improve the function of your thyroid, or get rid of the unpleasantness caused by the symptoms of your hypothyroidism, in that case, few bottles of essential oils is all you need.

Here are 5 natural and simple ways in which you can use essential oils to improve your hypothyroidism:

1.	By combining three drops of frankincense oil with 5 drops of clove oil and lemongrass oil each, you can improve your thyroid function. Simply rub this mixture at the lower part of your neck, directly on the thyroid, and let the oils work their magic. You can also gain get the same effect if you put 2 drops of frankincense oil in your mouth, two times each day.

2.	Combine one part of lemongrass oil and one part of myrrh oil. Apply 2-4 drops of this mixture on the thyroid area and rub the mixture with your fingers. You can also rub the same mixture on your wrists or the reflexology points on your big toes, for the same effect.

3.	If you have pain in your joints or muscles as a result of your hypothyroidism, then you can try relieving the pain by soaking in a soothing warm bath where you have put a couple of drops of each clove oil, myrrh, geranium, and lemongrass oil.

4. If you have been experiencing fatigue, you can easily combat it by adding a drop of peppermint and citrus oil in your hand. Cup your hand over your hand, and inhale.

5. If you have been irritable, anxious, and you wish to improve your mood, try using oils such as lavender, chamomile, and frankincense in your home diffuser.

The Next Step

Now that you know the exact steps that lead to the treatment of your underactive thyroid, the next step is to simply get rid of the foods and lifestyle habits that may disrupt its function and adopt a hypothyroid-friendly lifestyle and diet that will get rid of the onset of symptoms and complications and allow you to leave your life to the fullest.

One last thing! How awesome would it be if you shared your opinion about this book with a short review on Amazon? You read reviews yourself so why not give back a little to the community.

http://booksfor.review/lowthyroid

www.ingramcontent.com/pod-product-compliance
Lightning Source LLC
Chambersburg PA
CBHW030518290526
45786CB00004B/1510